Table of Contents

A headache is a pain in your head or face that's often described as a pressure that's throbbing, constant, sharp or dull. Headaches can differ greatly in regard to pain type, severity, location and frequency.

Headaches are a very common condition that most people will experience many times during their lives. They're the most common form of pain and are a major reason cited for days missed at work or school, as well as visits to healthcare providers.

While most headaches aren't dangerous, certain types can be a sign of a more serious condition.

BREAKFAST

1. Breakfast hash

Prep Time: 15 Minutes

Cook Time: 30 Minutes

Servings: 6

Ingredients

- 1 carrots
- 1 sweet potatoes
- 2 onions (green) scallions, spring onions
- 4 ounces mushrooms cremini or button
- 8 ounces tofu firm, extra-firm, super-firm
- 1/2 cup black beans cooked or canned (115 g)
- 1/4 head cabbage red or green (175 g)
- 1 stalk broccoli
- 3 cloves garlic
- 1/2-1 cup juicer pulp optional
- 2-4 tbsp Bragg's liquid aminos (or tamari)
- 2 tbsp sesame seeds

- 2-3 tsp dark toasted sesame oil
- 1-2 tsp hot chili oil

Instructions

1. Rinse and drain the beans. Wash all the vegetables, leaving the skins on.
2. Slice the mushrooms. Cut the carrot into thin diagonal slices. Thinly slice the cabbage. Cut the sweet potato into small dice (about ¼" cubes). Peel and mince the garlic cloves. Thinly slice the green onions or mince the sweet onion. Cut the broccoli into small chunks.
3. Heat about 2 T. olive or grapeseed oil in a large skillet or nonstick saute pan.
4. When the oil is shimmering, add the onions, carrots, mushrooms, and the sweet potato.
5. Cook, stirring every couple of minutes, for about ten minutes.
6. Break up the tofu with your fingers and add to the pot, along with the veggie pulp (if using).
7. Add the tamari, sesame oils, and sesame seeds.
8. Add the garlic, broccoli, beans, cabbage, and continue to cook for another five minutes.
9. Taste and adjust seasonings.

Prep Time: 30 Minutes

Cook Time: 35 Minutes

Servings: 16

Ingredients

- 4-8 ounces tempeh bacon optional
- 8 ounces mushrooms cremini
- 6 ounces onions yellow, 1 small or 1/2 large
- 10 ounces spinach fresh or frozen
- 3 cups milk soy, rice, almond, hemp
- 6 ounces tofu silken
- 3 tbsp flax seeds (ground)
- 1/2 tsp nutmeg (dried)
- 1/2 tsp black pepper
- 8 ounces cheddar (shredded, vegan) mozzarella flavor, or other vegan cheese
- 12 slices bread (gluten-free) cubed

Instructions

1. Oil an oven-proof casserole dish.

2. Preheat oven to 350F/180C/gas mark 4.

3. Mince the tempeh bacon and set aside.

4. Clean and thinly slice the mushrooms. Peel and mince the onions. Sauté onions and mushrooms in olive oil over medium heat until golden brown.

5. Squeeze the spinach dry if using frozen spinach.

6. Put the milk, tofu, flax seeds, nutmeg, and pepper in a blender or food processor and pulse just until blended.

7. In a large bowl, gently stir all ingredients until evenly mixed. Spread into the casserole dish.

8. Bake until golden and puffy, about 35-45 minutes. Let sit about ten minutes before cutting.

Prep Time: 20 Minutes

Cook Time: 50 Minutes

Servings: 12

Ingredients

- 1/2 cup butter (unsalted) can use vegan butter or Spectrum organic shortening
- 1 cup granulated sugar (organic)
- 2 eggs
- 1 teaspoon vanilla extract
- 2 cups all-purpose flour (gluten-free) Bob's Red Mill Gluten-Free 1 to 1 Baking Flour
- 1/2 teaspoon sea salt can omit for low-sodium version
- 1/2 teaspoon baking soda can use sodium-free baking soda
- 1/4 cup yogurt sour milk, buttermilk, or kefir
- 2 bananas ripe, mashed with a fork

Streusel mixture

- 1/2 cup brown sugar

- 2 tablespoons all-purpose flour (gluten-free) Bob's Red Mill Gluten-Free 1 to 1 Baking Flour
- 2 tablespoons butter (unsalted) melted
- 2 teaspoons cinnamon
- 1/2 cup walnuts finely chopped

Instructions

1. Preheat oven to 350F°/180C°/gas mark 4. Grease a 6 ½" by 10" cake pan (or similar size).
2. Cream butter and sugar in mixing bowl.
3. Add eggs & vanilla extract, beating until fluffy.
4. Sift dry ingredients together, then add to batter with yogurt and mashed bananas.
5. Put half of batter into prepared pan.
6. Combine streusel ingredients in a bowl and mix well. Sprinkle half over the batter in the pan.
7. Scrape in rest of the batter and smooth the top, then sprinkle over the rest of the streusel.
8. Bake for 35-50 minutes (will depend on the size of your pan). Top should be firm in the center and spring back when pressed with a finger, but be careful as the sugar in the streusel will be very hot.

9. Cool complete on a wire rack before cutting into squares.

Prep Time: 10 Minutes

Cook Time: 10 Minutes

Servings: 4

Ingredients

- 1/2 cup rice medium- or long-grain white rice
- 1 cup water (filtered or spring) plus 1 tablespoon for the eggs
- 6 eggs
- 4 tbsp grapeseed oil divided use
- 5 cloves garlic peeled and thinly sliced
- 3 stalks onions (green) white parts thinly sliced, green parts thinly sliced on the diagonal (separate use)
- 1 pound tomatoes ripe, skin removed, cut into wedges and de-seeded
- 1/4 tsp sea salt can omit for low-sodium, migraine, and Meniere's diet
- 1/2 tsp dark toasted sesame oil

Instructions

1. Rinse and strain the rice 3 times or until the water runs clear. Bring to a boil with the 1 cup of water in a saucepan with the lid on (this takes about 5 minutes over high heat). Turn down to low and cook for 13 minutes without stirring. Turn off the heat and let sit for 5 minutes with the lid on.

2. Beat the eggs with 1 tablespoon water in a bowl.

3. In a large non-stick frying pan or wok, heat 2 tablespoons of the grapeseed oil over high heat just until it begins to smoke. Scramble the eggs using a spatula to push them around, just until barely set, about 1 minute. Remove the eggs to a bowl and wipe out the pan.

4. Wipe out the pan, then add the remaining 2 tablespoons of the grapeseed oil and return to the heat. Add garlic and the white part of the green onions and saute about 1 minute, just until you smell the aromatics and they are starting to get some color.

5. Add the tomatoes and half the salt (if using). Cook until the tomatoes are starting to break down into a sauce.

6. Add the cooked eggs, breaking them up with a spatula as you stir. Add the remaining salt (if using) and the sesame oil.

7. Put into bowls with some of the steamed rice and garnish with the remaining green onion.

8. To blanch the tomatoes: Bring a medium-sized pot of water to a rolling bowl. Cut an X in the bottom of the tomato(es). Drop into the water and cook one minute. Remove with a slotted spoon, let cool, then slip off the skin. Core and cut into wedges, removing the seeds as you do so.

Prep Time: 2hrs 10 Minutes

Cook Time: 35 Minutes

Servings: 6

Ingredients

- Caramelized onions
- 5 onions yellow, brown, or white (not red)
- 1 tbsp olive oil (extra virgin)
- 1 tbsp butter (unsalted)
- 3/4 tsp kosher salt can omit for lower-sodium version
- 2 sprigs thyme (fresh)
- Caramelized onion tart
- 1 sheet puff pastry (gluten-free) Schar brand, thawed overnight in the fridge
- 1 tbsp Dijon mustard or mayonnaise
- 1 cup caramelized onions recipe here
- 1/3 cup olives (black) I used 4 olives total, thinly sliced, to reduce the sodium
- 8-10 anchovy fillets oil-packed, can omit

Instructions

Caramelized onions:

1. Cut the onions in half from stem to root end, peel, and thinly slice. Don't be perfect about it. Discard any tough root ends. Alternatively (saving time and tears), you can use the slicing disc on your food processor to slice peeled, quartered onions.
2. Heat a large heavy-bottomed pan (with an available lid) over medium-high heat. Add the olive oil and butter.
3. Once the butter is melted, add the onions. Stir. Add the salt and thyme. Keep stirring every few minutes. The onions will give off about a cup of liquid almost immediately.
4. When the onions have softened a bit and are starting to turn translucent (about 5 minutes), turn down the heat to low and throw on the lid. Cook, covered, stirring every 10 minutes or so, until the onions have turned very soft, translucent, and very sweet, and have released a good cup or two of juices, at least one hour and up to two.
5. If the onions start to brown, add a splash of water or chicken stock.

6. Remove the lid for good, turn the heat to medium-high, and bring to a gentle boil. Cook, stirring almost constantly, until nearly all the liquid in the pan has evaporated and the onions have taken on a marmalade-like consistency (golden yellow, honey-sweet, and still moist), about 15 minutes.Stay with it. Don't let it burn. Stir, stir, stir.

7. Locate the thyme sprigs and discard. Taste. Add salt if needed. Cool. The onions keep in a covered container for a few days in the fridge and for several months in the freezer.

8. Caramelized onion tart:

9. Take your tart dough out of the fridge or freezer. Once it's soft enough to roll out, preheat the oven to 350ºF.

10. Roll out your tart dough until it's about 10 inches in diameter and ⅛-inch thick. Press into an 8-or 9-inch tart pan. You can also do this as a free- form tart. [The Schar gluten-free pastry comes on a piece of parchment paper and is already 1/8" thick so just unroll it and put it on a baking pan, covering the entire crust in the next step.]

11. Thinly spread the mustard or mayonnaise over the puff pastry with a pastry brush or a butter knife. Spread a cup of the caramelized onions over the crust.

Top with olives and anchovies (if using) in any pattern that you like.

12. Bake until the crust is just set and the onions are golden brown, about 35 to 40 minutes. [You should be able to lift it up with a spatula and it's like a board, not sagging in the middle.]

13. Serve warm or at room temperature with a crisp green salad. Freezes beautifully.

Prep Time: 15 Minutes

Cook Time: 25 Minutes

Servings: 4

Ingredients

- 3 eggs egg replacer
- 3/4 cup milk soy, rice, hemp, coconut (rice, hemp, coconut for migraine diet)
- 3/4 cup all-purpose flour (gluten-free) (100 g)
- 1 tsp vanilla extract
- 1/4 tsp sea salt (omit for low-sodium and migraine diets)
- 2 pears apples, bananas (not bananas for migraine diet)
- 1 tbsp maple syrup maple sugar
- 3/4 tsp cinnamon
- 2 tbsp Earth Balance (unsalted butter for low-sodium and migraine diet)

Instructions

1. Preheat oven to 450F/230C/gas mark 7 and place a 12-inch cast iron skillet on the middle rack. You need a cast iron skillet for this to work, as it needs to be screaming hot when you put the ingredients in.In a medium bowl (or stand mixer), whisk together the first five ingredients.

2. Peel and core the fruit, slice thinly, and toss the fruit with the cinnamon and sugar in a separate bowl.

3. When the oven reaches temperature, remove the skillet using hot pads, place on a flat, heat-proof surface, and add the butter or margarine. Swirl the pan so that it is coated evenly and up the sides about an inch. Add the fruit and shake to distribute evenly. Pour the batter over the fruit. Don't worry if it floats.

4. Place the pan back in the oven and bake for 25 minutes until puffed and golden.

5. Serve with more margarine or butter and maple syrup.

Prep Time: 10 Minutes

Cook Time: 30 Minutes

Servings: 10

Ingredients

Crepes:

- 1/3 cup sweet sorghum flour (45 g)
- 1/4 cup tapioca flour (40 g)
- 1/4 cup brown rice flour (40 g)
- 1/4 cup teff flour or seeds (49 g)
- 1 cup milk organic, or half and half
- 1/4 cup water (filtered or spring)

3 eggs:

- 3 tbsp butter (unsalted) organic or Kerrygold
- Vanilla ricotta cream
- 15 ounces ricotta (whole-milk) organic
- 1 tbsp vanilla extract
- 1/2 tsp cinnamon Vietnamese if possible
- 1/8-1/4 tsp nutmeg (dried) freshly ground
- 2-3 packets stevia (organic) Pyure brand

Instructions

Crepes

1. Put the first four ingredients in the blender and blend until a fine powder.
2. Add milk, water, and eggs and blend for one minute. Let stand at least 20 minutes, 30 is better.
3. Melt the butter and blend in just before cooking the crepes.
4. Heat a non-stick large skillet or frying pan over medium heat. No oil is needed; there is enough in the batter.
5. Pulse once or twice to remix, each time, before pouring 1/4 cup of batter into the center of the pan, tilting it in a circle to spread the batter into a thin circle.
6. Cook two minutes until just set, then flip with a spatula or tongs, and cook another 30 seconds.
7. Remove to a plate, then pour the next crepe. I fill the ones we are going to eat while each is cooking, putting them on another plate.
8. Stuff with ricotta cream and berries.
9. Cool extra crepes on separate plates (they stick together), then stack, separated by waxed paper, and

wrap with plastic wrap, in a heavy freezer-safe bag to freeze. They are also great for dinner.

10. Vanilla ricotta cream

11. Mix together in a bowl, then replace back in the tub for storage. Eat within four days.

12. To fill crepes, put into a zip-top bag, close, then snip off a corner and use it to pipe the cream into each crepe.

Prep Time: 10 Minutes

Cook Time: 1hrs 30 Minutes

Servings: 6

Ingredients

- 1 cup corn grits (white, stone-ground) polenta 135 g (or one tube pre-cooked polenta, sliced)
- 2 tsp sea salt
- 1/2 tsp black pepper
- 25 ounces tomato sauce chunky spicy marinara (700 g)
- 3 bell peppers roasted (12 oz jar/240 g dry)
- 14 ounces artichoke hearts jarred or frozen
- 6 ounces spinach fresh, baby
- 1 cup mozzarella (shredded, vegan) (115 g)
- 1/2 cup pine nuts raw (75 g)
- 1 handful basil leaves (fresh)

Instructions

1. Heat 4 cups (1 L) of water in a large heavy-bottomed pot over high heat until boils. Slowly pour in the polenta while whisking constantly. Reduce the heat to low, cover and cook, stirring occasionally with a wooden spoon for about 20-30 minutes. You want it to be very thick.

2. Remove the polenta from the heat and add 2 t. of the salt and whisk thoroughly. Taste and season with additional cracked black pepper and more salt if needed.

3. While the polenta is cooking, preheat the oven to 375F/190C/gas mark 5. If you are roasting the peppers yourself, here is how to roast bell peppers.

4. In a large oven-proof skillet, start heating the tomato sauce. Add the vegetables as you finish prepping them:

5. Drain and roughly chop the roasted peppers. (Or, peel the cooled roasted peppers and roughly chop.)

6. Drain and quarter the artichoke hearts. (Thaw and drain frozen ones.)

7. Add the spinach about 10 minutes before you want to put the dish in the oven. Put a lid on the pan to help

the spinach wilt down. Stir everything gently to mix well.

8. Make a small well in the top of the tomato mixture and put a generous dollop of polenta in it. Repeat until you have about 6 polenta scoops on top. Or, place the sliced polenta across the top in a layer, nestling it down into the sauce so it's partially covered.

9. Sprinkle the polenta with the cheese and then the pine nuts.

10. Bake for 20-25 minutes until bubbly and the pine nuts are golden brown.

Prep Time: 10 Minutes

Cook Time: 15 Minutes

Servings: 4

Ingredients

French toast:

- 1 cup soy milk almond milk
- 2 tbsp coconut flour (10 g)
- 1 tbsp flax seeds (ground) (6 g)
- 1 tsp vanilla extract
- 1/2 tsp cinnamon highest quality, like Vietnamese
- 1/4 tsp nutmeg (dried) freshly grated if possible

Strawberry-kumquat compote

- 8 ounces kumquats
- 8 ounces strawberries
- 1/2 cup pecans raw (50 g)
- 2 tbsp agave syrup or honey
- 1 tbsp cassis (fruit vinegar)

Instructions

French toast

1. Grind the flax seeds in a blender or spice grinder. Whisk all the ingredients together in a shallow bowl and let sit a few minutes to thicken.
2. Heat a nonstick frying pan or griddle over medium heat until drops of water bounce off the top.
3. Spray with cooking spray (for cast iron) or use a neutral oil like canola or grapeseed oil just to coat the surface. (Do not using cooking spray on nonstick pans; it will ruin the surface.)
4. Place a slice of bread in the milk mixture and let soak in, then turn, allowing the other side to soak up the mixture. When the pan is hot, add the slice of bread and start soaking another.
5. Cook for 4 minutes on the first side, 3-4 minutes on the second side. Keep warm in the oven while you are cooking the rest.

Kumquat-strawberry compote

1. Prepare the kumquats by washing well to remove any waxy coating (if store-bought). Home-grown kumquats just need a rinse. Trim off the ends of the kumquats, then stand up on one cut end and slice

lengthwise. Peel the inner flesh and white pith away from the peel. Compost the flesh and pith; you will use only the peel, which is sweet. For a great step-by-step demo, see Recipe Girl's kumquat marmalade post.

2. Thinly slice the peels and place in a bowl.
3. Hull the strawberries using a paring knife to trim out the white center under the green leaves. Compost the tops. Thinly slice the strawberries. Tip: If you stand them cut side down it's easier to slice them lengthwise. Add to the bowl.
4. Roughly chop the pecans and add to the bowl.
5. Whisk the agave syrup and vinegar together, then pour over the fruit, tossing lightly.

Prep Time: 10 Minutes

Cook Time: 30 Minutes

Servings: 16

Ingredients

- 1-1/2 cups cornbread mix (gluten-free) (265 g)
- 2-1/4 cups corn frozen, divided, no salt added (300 g)
- 1/4 cup agave syrup maple syrup, honey
- 1/4 cup grapeseed oil sunflower, olive oil
- 1-1/4 cups water (filtered or spring)

Instructions

1. Preheat oven to 350°F. Grease a 9" x 13" pan or prepare muffin cups.
2. Put 1 cup of corn in the blender with the agave syrup, oil, and water. Blend until fairly smooth.
3. Mix with remaining ingredients and pour into prepared pan. Bake casserole for about 30 minutes or until the top springs back in the center when touched

with a finger. If making this in muffin tins, check after
20 minutes.

11. Merguez Turkey Sausage Patties

Prep Time: 10 Minutes

Cook Time: 10 Minutes

Servings: 16

Ingredients

- 16 ounces turkey (ground)
- 2 cloves garlic
- 1/2 cup Italian flat-leaf parsley (fresh) or cilantro leaves
- 1-1/2 tsp smoked paprika
- 1 tsp fennel (dried) ground
- 1 tsp cumin (dried)
- 1/2 tsp coriander (dried)
- 1/2 tsp cream of tartar
- 1/4 tsp baking soda omit for lowest-sodium version
- 1/4 tsp smoked salt omit for lowest-sodium version
- 1 pinch cinnamon
- 1 pinch cayenne pepper
- 1 pinch black pepper

Instructions

1. Place parsley and garlic in a food processor and process until finely minced. Add meat and sprinkle in remaining ingredients, then pulse just until blended.
2. Heat extra virgin olive oil in a non-stick pan over medium heat. Form patties straight from the food processor using an ice cream scoop, flattening them as you add them to the hot oil.
3. Cook about 3 minutes per side, until meat is cooked through.
4. Serve immediately, refrigerate to use later, or freeze once completely cool.

Prep Time: 10 Minutes

Cook Time: 10 Minutes

Servings: 12

Ingredients

- 1 head cabbage green or Savoy
- 1 carrots large
- 2 onions (green) scallions, spring onions
- 1/4 cup dark toasted sesame oil
- 1/4 cup rice wine vinegar
- 1 piece ginger (fresh) 1" or about the size of your first knuckle
- 1-3 cloves garlic see notes
- 2 tbsp sesame seeds black or tan

Instructions

1. Wash the cabbage and the scallions and shake them dry. Using a sharp paring knife, cut out the core of the cabbage.

2. Shred the cabbage using a food processor, or slice thinly with a large sharp knife.

3. Chop the scallions into small pieces.

4. Put a skillet on medium heat and warm it up. Add the sesame seeds to the dry skillet and toast them until golden brown or they start to pop. If using black sesame seeds, watch for the popping and remove them before they burn.

5. Over a very large bowl, use a Microplane zester or fine grater to grate the ginger. Press or finely grate the garlic cloves and add them to the bowl. If the garlic cloves are large, just use one. At certain times of year the heads of garlic are tiny, so I used three mini cloves.

6. I usually mince garlic, but I do like a garlic press when adding garlic to a dressing, as it gives you juice and fine bits. You can also press slices of fresh ginger through a garlic press.

7. Pour in the oil and vinegar and whisk together. Add the cabbage, carrots, and scallions and toss until evenly coated. Sprinkle with the sesame seeds and refrigerate.

Prep Time: 15 Minutes

Cook Time: 50 Minutes

Servings: 10

Ingredients

- 1 pound dried beans SOAKED OVERNIGHT in filtered or spring water. I used a 10-bean blend. Use any of these for the migraine diet: chickpeas, white beans, kidney beans, split peas, black beans,
- 2 tbsp olive oil (extra virgin)
- 1 onions diced. Use a bunch of green onions for the migraine diet.
- 2 cloves garlic minced
- 2 carrots peeled and sliced into coins
- 2 potatoes new or Yukon gold (but any type will do), large dice
- 4 ounces beef (grass-fed) pork or lamb, cubed (can omit to make this vegan)
- 4 cups water (filtered or spring)
- 1/4 cup tomato paste or red pepper paste/puree
- 3 bay leaves

- 3 thyme (fresh) 2-3 sprigs
- 1 tbsp Italian seasoning salt-free OR Porcini Paradiso from Spice Tribe

Instructions

1. Soak the dried beans overnight in plenty of water. If possible, use filtered or spring water for the best flavor. Rinse and drain.
2. Heat the oil in the Instant Pot set to Saute (medium heat level). Saute the onion, garlic, and carrots for 5 minutes or until turning golden.
3. Add the Italian seasoning and cook for 1 minute to release the oils.
4. Add remaining ingredients and stir well, making sure the tomato paste is dissolved. Hit Cancel.
5. Secure the lid, then set to Pressure Cook on high for 25 minutes. Use natural pressure release. After opening the lid, remove the 3 bay leaves and the thyme sprigs. Serve hot, garnished with more fresh thyme if desired.

Prep Time: 15 Minutes

Cook Time: 30 Minutes

Servings: 8

Ingredients

Salad:

- 2 tbsp olive oil (extra virgin)
- 1 onions small red, finely diced
- 2 carrots peeled and finely diced
- 1 stalk celery finely diced
- 1-1/2 cups lentils preferably French green
- 3 cups chicken stock (low-sodium) use vegetable stock to make this vegetarian/vegan
- 1 bay leaves
- 1 clove garlic smashed and peeled
- 1 cup walnuts lightly toasted and chopped (can omit or serve on the side for people with nut allergies)
- 1 lemons juiced

- 4 ounces feta cheese crumbled (omit for vegan version)
- 1/4 cup Italian flat-leaf parsley (fresh) minced

Dressing:

- 1 shallots finely minced
- 1 tsp Dijon mustard
- 2 tbsp red wine vinegar or sherry vinegar
- 1/3 cup olive oil (extra virgin)
- 1 tsp kosher salt use less if watching your sodium
- 1 tsp black pepper

Instructions

1. Pour the olive oil into the inner pot of your electric pressure cooker. Select the Saute function and set the heat level to "Normal." When the oil is shimmering, after about 2 minutes, add the onion, carrots, and celery and saute until softened, about 5 minutes. Using a slotted spoon, remove the vegetables to a large serving bowl and set aside. Press Cancel to turn off the Saute function.
2. Add the lentils, broth, bay leaf, and garlic. Close the lid and make sure the pressure release valve is closed.

Select the Pressure Cook function and set the cooking time to 9 minutes at high pressure.

3. Make the dressing: In a small bown, whisk together the shallot, mustard, and vinegar. While whisking, slowly add the oil in a steady stream and continue whisking until emulsified. Add the salt and pepper to taste.

4. When the cooking program is complete, release the pressure manually and remove the lid. Drain the lentils, discarding the bay leaf, and add them to the bowl with the cooked vegetables. Add the dressing to the lentils while they are still warm and stir to combine.

5. Let the lentils cool to room temperature before adding the walnuts, lemon juice, feta, and parsley. Taste and adjust the seasoning, adding more salt and pepper if necessary. Serve at room temperature.

Prep Time: 15 Minutes

Cook Time: 30 Minutes

Servings: 8

Ingredients

Salad:

- 2 tbsp olive oil (extra virgin)
- 1 onions small red, finely diced
- 2 carrots peeled and finely diced
- 1 stalk celery finely diced
- 1-1/2 cups lentils preferably French green
- 3 cups chicken stock (low-sodium) use vegetable stock to make this vegetarian/vegan
- 1 bay leaves
- 1 clove garlic smashed and peeled
- 1 cup walnuts lightly toasted and chopped (can omit or serve on the side for people with nut allergies)
- 1 lemons juiced

- 4 ounces feta cheese crumbled (omit for vegan version)
- 1/4 cup Italian flat-leaf parsley (fresh) minced

Dressing:

- 1 shallots finely minced
- 1 tsp Dijon mustard
- 2 tbsp red wine vinegar or sherry vinegar
- 1/3 cup olive oil (extra virgin)
- 1 tsp kosher salt use less if watching your sodium
- 1 tsp black pepper

Instructions

1. Pour the olive oil into the inner pot of your electric pressure cooker. Select the Saute function and set the heat level to "Normal." When the oil is shimmering, after about 2 minutes, add the onion, carrots, and celery and saute until softened, about 5 minutes. Using a slotted spoon, remove the vegetables to a large serving bowl and set aside. Press Cancel to turn off the Saute function.
2. Add the lentils, broth, bay leaf, and garlic. Close the lid and make sure the pressure release valve is closed.

Select the Pressure Cook function and set the cooking time to 9 minutes at high pressure.

3. Make the dressing: In a small bown, whisk together the shallot, mustard, and vinegar. While whisking, slowly add the oil in a steady stream and continue whisking until emulsified. Add the salt and pepper to taste.

4. When the cooking program is complete, release the pressure manually and remove the lid. Drain the lentils, discarding the bay leaf, and add them to the bowl with the cooked vegetables. Add the dressing to the lentils while they are still warm and stir to combine.

5. Let the lentils cool to room temperature before adding the walnuts, lemon juice, feta, and parsley. Taste and adjust the seasoning, adding more salt and pepper if necessary. Serve at room temperature.

Prep Time: 30 Minutes

Cook Time: 30 Minutes

Servings: 12

Ingredients

- 2 cups spinach packed, then finely chopped (90 g)
- 1 onions red, diced
- 1 2-inch ginger (fresh) peeled, then minced or grated
- 1-3 hot chiles (Habañero or similar) fresh Thai, serrano, or cayenne, stemmed, seeded, minced
- 1 cup chickpea flour gram, besan flour (110g)
- 1 teaspoon sea salt omit for low-sodium diet
- 1 teaspoon red chile powder or cayenne (can adjust if you need less heat)
- 1/2 teaspoon turmeric (dried)
- 1/2 teaspoon aijwan (carom seeds)
- 1/2 cup water (filtered or spring) warm. Start with 1/4 cup and see how the batter sets up.
- 2 cups grapeseed oil for frying

Instructions

1. In a large mixing bowl, combine the spinach, onion, ginger, and fresh chiles and mix well to combine. Set aside.

2. In a separate large mixing bowl, combine the besan, salt, red chile powder, turmeric, and ajwain and stir well to combine. You can also add other spices, including garam masala, ground black pepper, and so on. Be as creative as you like. Add half the water to the besan mixture and stir until smooth. This mixture should be fairly thick and not too watery. Make sure that there are no lumps in the batter.

3. Slowly fold the spinach mixture into the batter.

4. Ina small kadhai, wok, or saucepan over medium–high heat, warm the oil. The oil should be about 1 inch / 3 cm deep in the deepest part of the kadhai. You'll know the oil is hot enough if you drop in a cumin seed and it sizzles and rises to the top immediately. You're looking for 350-360F if you have an instant-read thermometer.

5. Using a tablespoon measure, carefully place 4 tablespoons / 60 mL of batter into the oil, 1 at a time, and cook for about 30 seconds on 1 side, until lightly browned but just shy of being cooked through. Turn

over each of the pakoras and cook for 30 seconds more.

6. Remove the pakoras with a slotted spoon and transfer to a baking sheet lined with a paper towel to absorb extra oil. Place a small, flat bowl on top of each pakora and press down lightly.

7. Return the pakoras to the hot oil and cook for 30 to 40 seconds on each side, until golden brown. Remove from the heat. Remove the pakoras with a slotted spoon and transfer to the baking tray lined with fresh paper towels to absorb the oil. on doing this to ensure the pakoras are extra crispy. It also helps to make sure they cook through. Don't worry: You can fry them just once as well. Just cook them a little longer to ensure they cook through.] I cooked mine for 2-3 minutes per side, until golden brown and puffed up.

8. Cook remaining batter in the same way until all are cooked. Eat immediately. These are normally served with Mint or Tamarind-Date Chutney.

Prep Time: 15 Minutes

Cook Time: 35 Minutes

Servings: 6

Ingredients

- 3/4 cup white rice japonica (sushi)
- 8 cups water (filtered or spring) plus 2 tbsp for chicken marinade
- 12 ounces chicken breast partially frozen then sliced as thinly as you can
- 2 tsp cornstarch organic if possible (so no GMOs)
- 1 tbsp oyster sauce (gluten-free version)
- 1.5 tsp chicken bouillon divided use, optional
- 2 tbsp grapeseed oil or other neutral vegetable oil
- 1 knob ginger (fresh) peeled and cut into thinnest matchsticks
- 2 green onions thinly sliced on the diagonal
- 1/4 cup cilantro stems only, finely chopped
- 1 tsp sea salt

Instructions

1. Wash and drain rice three times.

2. Bring 8 cups of water to a boil on high heat.

3. Combine thinly sliced chicken, cornstarch, oyster sauce, 2 tablespoons additional water, 1/2 teaspoon bouillon (if using), and 2 tablespoons vegetable oil in a bowl, mixing with your hands until the chicken is well-coated. Set aside.

4. Once the water in the big pot is at a rolling bowl, stir in the rice. Don't stir the rice once it's back to a boil as it's more likely to stick to the bottom of the pot. Once it's come back to a boil, partially cover and turn down to medium heat. It should have bubbles breaking the surface but not be actively boiling. Cook for 25 minutes without touching the pan.

5. Remove cover and begin whisking the rice rapidly and constantly for about 3 minutes, until the rice breaks down and the liquid thickens into a porridge consistency.

6. Turn up the heat to boiling again and add the chicken in small amounts while stirring constantly, so the chicken doesn't clump together. It should all be cooked through in 2-3 minutes. Check to make sure the chicken is fully cooked before turning off the heat.

7. Taste. You can add (optional) up to 1 teaspoon sea salt and one more teaspoon chicken bouillon (per Made with Lau). Stir in the ginger.

8. Ladle into bowls and top with cilantro and green onions. Additional traditional toppings include chopped salted peanuts, Chinese salted fish, Chinese preserved vegetables.

Prep Time: 10 Minutes

Cook Time: 20 Minutes

Servings: 12

Ingredients

- 15.5 ounces kidney beans red, cooked, no salt added
- 15.5 ounces wax beans cooked, no salt added
- 15.5 ounces chickpeas garbanzo beans, cooked, no salt added
- 1 potatoes red, can add more
- 1 onions (green) finely chopped

Dressing:

- 1/2 cup apple cider or apple juice
- 1/4 cup olive oil (extra virgin)
- 2 tablespoon white vinegar use apple cider vinegar once you have tested it on the Plan
- 1 tsp sea salt fine, omit for low-sodium diets
- 1 tsp white pepper finely ground
- 1 packet stevia (organic) powdered, or liquid stevia to equal 1 teaspoon sugar, optional

Instructions

Salad:

1. Rinse the beans well and leave in the colander to drain while you make the rest of the dish.
2. Dice the scrubbed potatoes finely. Rinse three times to remove the starch. Add filtered water just to cover and cook for 10 minutes until fork tender. I cook them in a microwave-safe dish, but you could boil them too. Drain immediately and rinse with cold water.
3. Finely chop the green onion and add to a cup of cold water for a few minutes to remove the bite. Drain well.

Dressing:

1. Add the apple cider or juice to a small saucepan set over medium heat. Bring to a boil, then reduce the heat to low and simmer for about 10 minutes, or until the liquid is reduced to 2 tablespoons. Remove from the heat and let cool.
2. Put all the dressing ingredients in a jar, and shake well to emulsify. Toss all the ingredients together in a large bowl and pour over about half of the dressing. Toss well; the flavors will intensify as it marinates. Refrigerate up to 5 days. Use leftover dressing on salads.

Prep Time: 20 Minutes

Cook Time: 1hrs 20 Minutes

Servings: 12

Ingredients

- 2 tbsp olive oil (extra virgin) or ghee (use olive oil for plant-based diet)
- 1 onion diced (use 2 bunches green onions for migraine and low-tyramine diet)
- 1 tbsp curry powder mild or medium (salt-free version)
- 1 tbsp nigella seeds optional
- 1 tbsp mustard seeds optional
- 1 cup lentils (use yellow split peas or chana dal for migraine and low-tyramine diets)
- 4 cups vegetable stock (low-sodium) can use low-sodium chicken broth
- 1 cup cabbage shredded, or spicy cabbage slaw
- 1/4 cup cilantro minced or Italian flat-leaf parsley if you hate cilantro

Instructions

1. Heat oil or ghee in large Dutch oven over medium heat until shimmering. Sauté onion until golden brown, about 5 minutes.
2. Sprinkle curry powder and seeds over the mixture (if using) and cook for 1 minute more or until seeds start popping.
3. Stir in lentils, broth, and cabbage and bring to a boil. Turn down and simmer for 30-60 minutes until lentils are very tender. (Time will vary based on type and age of lentil.)
4. Stir in minced herbs and serve by itself or over cooked basmati rice. This freezes beautifully.

Prep Time: 20 Minutes

Cook Time: 20 Minutes

Servings: 10

Ingredients

- 2 bunches Italian flat-leaf parsley (fresh) can substitute curly parsley (use stems)
- 1 bunch mint leaves (fresh) remove stems
- 2 onions (green) scallions, spring onions
- 16 ounces cherry tomatoes
- 1 cucumbers English, organic if possible, or 4 Persian cucumbers, diced
- 5.64ounces hemp seeds shelled (also called hemp hearts), 1 cup
- 1 lemon juiced (substitute 2 teaspoons organic white vinegar for migraine diet)
- 2 tablespoons olive oil (extra virgin)
- 1/2 teaspoon black pepper
- 1/2 teaspoon sea salt omit for migraine and low-sodium diets

Instructions

1. Use a food processor with the S-blade to chop the parsley and mint leaves, working in batches. Pulse on short blasts, about 5 pulses, until the leaves are chopped and most of the stems are not visible. Add to a large serving bowl.

2. Add the tomatoes to the food processor and pulse about 10 times until they are roughly chopped. Add to the bowl.

3. Thinly slice the onions and add. Dice the cucumbers and add.

4. Add remaining ingredients and toss together. Refrigerate until ready to serve so the flavors meld.

21. Paleo Dirty Rice

Prep Time: 10 Minutes

Cook Time: 40 Minutes

Servings: 6

Ingredients

- 2 tbsp olive oil (extra virgin) or rendered high-quality bacon fat
- 1-1/2 cups celery diced, with leaves (about 4 stalks)
- 2 cloves garlic
- 2 bell peppers red, diced
- 16 ounces turkey chorizo Diestel Farms
- 3 cups cauliflower (riced)
- 16 ounces kale or Swiss chard, chopped
- 2 tbsp cilantro can sub fresh Italian flat-leaf parsley if you hate cilantro
- 1/2 cup chicken stock (low-sodium) (if dry)

Instructions

1. Heat the oil in a large Dutch oven over medium heat until shimmering.
2. Sauté the celery for five minutes until softening and golden. Add the garlic, bell peppers and cook for 1 minute.
3. Add the turkey and cook, breaking up, for 5 minutes.
4. Add the remaining ingredients and cook for 25 minutes until the flavors are melded.
5. Serve at once. This freezes well and makes excellent lunches or dinners.

Prep Time: 20 Minutes

Cook Time: 1hrs 40 Minutes

Servings: 12

Ingredients

Ratatouille:

- 2 bunches onions (green) scallions, spring onions
- 4 tbsp olive oil (extra virgin) divided
- 4 cloves garlic thinly sliced
- 2 eggplants diced (aubergines)
- 2 zucchini diced (courgettes)
- 2 bell peppers red and yellow (capsicum), seeded and diced
- 4 tomatoes plum, or 8-12 cherry tomatoes
- 2-3 sprigs thyme (fresh)
- 1 handful basil leaves (fresh)
- Roasted spaghetti squash
- 1 spaghetti squash

Ground beef

- 32 ounces beef (grass-fed, ground) grass-fed

- 4 cloves garlic minced
- 1 tsp black pepper

Instructions

Ratatouille:

1. Heat 1 tbsp olive oil in a large cast iron or nonstick pan over medium-high heat. Sauté the onions until they are soft.
2. Add the garlic and cook until soft.
3. Transfer to a deep roasting pan or oven-safe baking dish.
4. Sauté each of the other vegetables separately, adding more oil as needed, until each is golden.
5. Transfer as you finish to the baking dish.
6. Add the tomatoes, uncooked, and thyme, and season with a tiny amount of salt and a generous amount of black pepper. Drizzle with additional olive oil. Stir to combine.
7. Bake at 350F/180C/gas mark 4 for about 40 minutes until soft and tender.
8. Stir in a handful of torn basil leaves before serving.

Roasted spaghetti squash

1. Wash one squash. Slice off each end, then slice lengthwise.

2. Use a spoon (grapefruit spoons work great for this) to scrape out the seeds and stringy bits. Spray or oil the cut side of the squash, then place cut side down on a baking sheet lined with parchment paper or a silicone liner.

3. Roast at 350F/180C/gas mark 4 for 35-45 minutes until fork tender.

4. Let cool enough to handle.

5. Use a fork to separate the flesh into spaghetti-like strands. Compost or toss the skin.

Ground beef

1. Heat 1 tbsp coconut oil over medium-high heat in a cast-iron frying pan or non-stick pan. (You can use the pan you sautéed the vegetables in.)

2. Add grass-fed ground beef and garlic.

3. Add a tiny amount of salt and a generous amount of black pepper.

4. Sauté the beef until cooked through and no longer pink.

5. Pour off or blot up any excess fat with a paper towel; reserve in a glass jar for another use. (Saturated fat is

key for migraine brains and is fine to eat so long as you keep your sugar and flour intake low.)

6. Add the ratatouille to the beef and cook until all flavors are combined.

7. Serve over warm spaghetti squash strands and a side salad (shown). Garnish with fresh thyme.

Prep Time: 30 Minutes

Cook Time: 45 Minutes

Servings: 8

Ingredients

Casserole:

- 8 ounces pasta (gluten-free) radiatore or rotini
- 4 cups kale finely shredded (100 g)
- 8 ounces soy chorizo (or quinrizo)
- 2 pieces corn bread 3 ounces (about 90 g)

Cashew cheez sauce

- 1/2 cup cashew butter (130 g)
- 3 tbsp lemon juice (fresh)
- 3 tbsp nutritional yeast
- 1-1/2 tbsp miso light or chickpea
- 1 tsp onion powder
- 1 pinch garlic powder
- 1 cup water (filtered or spring)

Instructions

Casserole:

1. Preheat the oven to 350F/180C/gas mark 4.
2. Cook the pasta according to package directions, usually about 10 minutes. Make sure you use a big pot, a lot of water, and have it really boiling. I add a good spoonful of salt and a small splash of olive oil, which seems to help the gluten-free pasta's consistency.
3. Finely shred the kale after removing the tough stems. Saute the kale with the soy chorizo in a skillet with a small amount of oil while the pasta is cooking.
4. After taste-testing the pasta to make sure it's just cooked through but not too soft, drain in a colander and rinse with cold water. Drain well.

Make the Cashew Cheez Sauce:

1. Spray a heatproof casserole dish with cooking spray. Toss the pasta with the kale-chorizo mixture (I use the rinsed-out pasta pan for this), then pour over the cheez sauce. Toss until everything is well-coated. Pour into the prepared casserole dish.
2. Crumble the stale cornbread into crumbs, making an even layer on top.

3. Bake for 30 minutes until the top is golden brown. Finely chop some fresh cilantro and sprinkle over the top.

4. Cashew cheez sauce

5. Place all ingredients in the blender except the water and blend until a smooth consistency. Add water until you get a thin pourable sauce. It will thicken as it bakes, so don't make it too thick.

Prep Time: 10 Minutes

Cook Time: 30 Minutes

Servings: 4

Ingredients

- 1 bunch Italian flat-leaf parsley (fresh)
- 1 sheet nori optional
- 3 cloves garlic large
- 1 tbsp sea salt kosher salt
- 8 ounces pasta (gluten-free) spaghetti
- 2 tbsp olive oil (extra virgin)
- 14 ounces tomatoes Italian plum, no salt added
- 1-1/2 cups olives (black) pitted, sliced (120 g)
- 4 tbsp capers (60 g)

Instructions

1. Pre-wash and spin dry the parsley.
2. If using, cut up the nori into tiny pieces using kitchen shears and set aside.

3. Smash the garlic cloves under the flat blade of a large chef's knife and remove the papery skin. Finely mince the garlic.

4. Bring a large pot of water to a boil, covered, and add 1 T. (5 g) kosher or sea salt.

5. Add the pasta to the boiling water, bring back to a boil, and add a few drops of olive oil to keep it from sticking. Using a wooden spoon keeps the pasta intact. Stir frequently with a wooden spoon, and cook until al dente.

6. Before draining, remove about 1/4 C. (60 ml) of pasta water to add to the sauce. The starch from the pasta water helps the sauce cling to the pasta.

7. Drain the pasta and rinse briefly with cold water. Drizzle with a little olive oil, shaking the colander to drain the water and stirring to coat the strands.

8. While the water is coming to a boil and you are cooking the pasta: Add olive oil to a large skillet or saute pan on medium heat. Once the oil is shimmering, turn down the heat to medium-low, adding the garlic and the minced nori. Cook, stirring frequently, until the garlic is golden brown, about 5 minutes.

9. Add the tomatoes, olives, and capers, stir well. Turn up the heat to medium. Cook the sauce until the pasta is done.

10. Add the drained pasta to the sauce.

11. Finely chop the parsley, then toss with the pasta.

25. Utica Greens

Prep Time: 10 Minutes

Cook Time: 30 Minutes

Servings: 8

Ingredients

Greens:

- 1 cup bacon (coconut) divided
- 1 tbsp olive oil (extra virgin)
- 5 cloves garlic peeled and minced
- 1-1/4 tsp red pepper flakes divided
- 1 bell peppers red, large, cored, seeded, and sliced into strips
- 12 ounces escarole pre-washed and chopped

Topping:

- 1 slice bread (gluten-free) toasted until very dry, torn into pieces
- 1 tbsp pine nuts
- 1 clove garlic peeled
- 1 tsp oregano (dried)
- 1 tsp basil (dried)

Instructions

1. Heat the oil over medium-high heat in a cast-iron (or oven-proof) skillet until shimmering. Add the garlic and hot pepper flakes and saute 30 seconds.
2. Add the peppers and saute 2-3 minutes.
3. Add half the coconut bacon and then the escarole (the pan will be very full). Put on the lid and cook for 15 minutes, stirring every 5 minutes as the escarole wilts.

Topping

1. Put the topping ingredients, including the remaining coconut bacon, in the food processor. Pulse until everything is uniform fine crumbs.
2. Turn on the broiler and place the rack just below it. When the escarole is nicely cooked, taste the dish. Add a little salt or more hot pepper flakes if it needs it. Sprinkle the topping evenly across the pan and broil for 3-5 minutes until golden brown. Serve at once.

Prep Time: 10 Minutes

Cook Time: 10 Minutes

Servings: 4

Ingredients

- 8 lamb loin chops about 1-1-1/2" thick
- 0.4 ounces mint leaves (fresh) 1/4 cup, packed leaves (no stems)
- 0.4 ounces Italian flat-leaf parsley (fresh) 1/4 cup, packed leaves (no stems)
- 0.4 ounces basil leaves (fresh) 1/4 cup, packed leaves (no stems)
- 1/2 cup olive oil (extra virgin)
- 1/4 cup white vinegar use white balsamic if not following the migraine diet
- 2 cloves garlic peeled, roughly chopped
- 1/2 tsp white pepper can substitute black pepper, but white is preferred
- 1/4 tsp red pepper flakes

Instructions

1. Put the meat out to warm up for at least 30 minutes before grilling.
2. Pulse all the other ingredients in a blender until emulsified. You should still see flecks of individual ingredients in the sauce.
3. Pour a small amount of sauce over the meat and rub on all sides. Marinate at least 30 minutes.
4. Heat a grill pan to high.
5. Sear the chops on high for 3 minutes per side, then 1 minute on each edge for a total of 10 minutes. (If using thinner chops, it should be about 6 minutes total.)
6. Use an instant-read thermometer; the internal temperature should be 130F/55C. Remove from heat and let rest 10 minutes before cutting. It should be medium-rare.
7. Serve with the rest of the sauce. In the photograph I included steamed rainbow carrots drizzled with olive oil.

Prep Time: 20 Minutes

Cook Time: 35 Minutes

Servings: 8

Ingredients

Crispy tofu sticks

- 16 ounces tofu super-firm or extra-firm, pressed
- 1/2 cup barbecue sauce recipe below
- 1/4 cup garbanzo bean flour chickpea flour, almond meal
- 1 tbsp nutritional yeast
- 1/2 tsp smoked salt
- 1 pinch white pepper optional
- 1/8 tsp garlic powder
- 1/8 tsp tsp onion powder
- Kid-friendly BBQ sauce
- 1/4 onions red, small, roughly chopped
- 1 tbsp olive oil (extra virgin)
- 1 tbsp apple cider vinegar
- 1 tbsp maple syrup organic

- 2 tbsp Bragg's liquid aminos (or tamari)
- 1 cup tomato sauce no salt added

Instructions

Crispy tofu sticks:

1. Press the tofu for at least 30 minutes (overnight if possible) using weights or a TofuXpress. If using weights, wrap the tofu in a clean kitchen towel and place between two cutting boards. Put a heavy frying pan or pile of cookbooks on top. Pressing the tofu removes more water from it, giving it a meatier texture and allowing it to absorb more flavor.
2. Cut the tofu into 16 sticks, using the short side as your length, and making the pieces as even as possible.
3. Prick the pieces all over with a fork to help the tofu absorb the marinade.
4. Put some of the barbecue sauce in the bottom of your marinating dish (something with a tight-fitting lid), add the tofu sticks, then pour the rest of the sauce over. Cover, shake well, and marinate in the refrigerator, overnight if possible.
5. Preheat the oven to 350F/180C/gas mark 4. Line a cookie sheet with parchment paper.

6. Mix the dry ingredients together in a shallow bowl, stirring with a fork. Take each piece of tofu and wipe off extra sauce with your fingers. Roll each piece of tofu in the breading, making sure it sticks to each side evenly and isn't too thick.

7. It should be a nice even coating. Place on the prepared cookie sheet. Spray with cooking spray, and flip over, making sure all the breading is thoroughly coated with spray. (If it's too thick then you need to add more spray.)

8. Bake for 15 minutes, then flip all the pieces over. Lightly spray any dry patches with more cooking spray. Bake another 18-20 minutes, until the sticks are crispy and golden brown. Serve with barbecue sauce, ranch dressing, or ketchup.

BBQ sauce

1. Sauté the onion in the oil over medium heat until golden, about 10 minutes. Add the remaining ingredients and simmer for 10 minutes. Puree in a blender until smooth.

Prep Time: 10 Minutes

Cook Time: 1hrs 35 Minutes

Servings: 8

Ingredients

Turkey:

- 1.4 pounds turkey breast (bone-in, skin on) (this was a small half-breast)
- .75 pounds turkey thigh (bone-in, skin on) (this was a much smaller thigh)

Dry rub:

- 1 tsp garlic powder
- 1/2 tsp thyme (dried)
- 1/4 tsp sea salt smoked if you have it (omit for salt-free diet)
- 1/4 tsp white pepper
- 1/4 tsp sage (dried)
- Pan gravy
- 4 tbsp brown rice flour use arrowroot starch or tapioca starch for paleo and Whole30 diets

- cups chicken stock (low-sodium) or homemade turkey stock
- 8 ounces mushrooms thinly sliced, optional

Instructions

How to roast turkey breast:

1. Let the turkey sit out until it's room temperature.
2. Preheat the oven to 350F/180C/gas mark 4. Place a rack in the center of the oven. While many online recipes call for starting the meat at 450F, and I do so for whole birds, I find that this can dry out smaller cuts of meat.
3. Prepare the roasting pan: Lightly spray or oil the rack, or create a "rack" by crumpling up a length of aluminum foil and creating a U-shape with it to keep the meat off the bottom of the pan.
4. Finely grind the dry rub ingredients together in a mortar and pestle or spice grinder. If you have meat totaling more than 2.25 pounds, double the dry rub amounts.
5. Use your fingers to work the rub under the skin and on the underside of the meat.
6. How to roast a turkey breast | Recipe Renovator

7. When you have coated the meat, stretch the skin over the meat as best you can. This creates a protective coating of fat that bastes the meat as it cooks.

8. How to roast a turkey breast | Recipe Renovator

9. Place the meat skin side up on the rack or foil rack, and place pan in the oven.

10. How to roast a turkey breast | Recipe Renovator

11. Set the timer for one hour, then check with a meat thermometer at the thickest part of the meat, but not hitting bone. Remove the turkey when it reaches 165F/75C. If you are cooking two pieces of meat, one will likely be done before the other. If it's close to 165F, check every five minutes. If it's not close (like 125F), set the timer for 10 minutes and check again. This is why an instant-read thermometer is super helpful. A large breast (4-6 pounds) may take 2 hours.

12. How to roast a turkey breast | Recipe Renovator

13. Remove turkey pieces to a cutting board and let rest 10 minutes. Note that turkey thigh meat is naturally pink, and may not look completely done because of this even if it has reached temperature. When in doubt, cut into the meat to the bone and see if it's completely cooked through. Remove skin and, if no

one in your group wants to eat it, save it for making stock with the bones.

14. How to roast a turkey breast | Recipe Renovator

Pan gravy

1. Once the turkey pieces are cooked, you can make pan gravy by putting the pan on the burners on medium heat. Make sure you use hot pads every time if moving an all-stainless steel pan like this one. Those handles are HOT.

2. If you want mushroom gravy, sauté the mushrooms in the pan drippings until golden, about 8 minutes. If the pan drippings are very dry, I mince up some of the turkey skin and cook that to release more fat. If cooking mushrooms and it's very dry, add some olive oil or other healthy fat.

3. Sprinkle 4 tablespoons brown rice flour into the pan drippings.

4. How to make turkey pan gravy | Recipe Renovator

5. Begin to stir the flour into the pan drippings, which in this case were quite dry.

6. How to make turkey pan gravy | Recipe Renovator

7. Once the flour is golden, add about 1/2 cup of the warm or hot chicken stock.

8. How to make turkey pan gravy | Recipe Renovator

9. Stir and cook into a roux (thick paste) for about five minutes until golden.

10. How to make turkey pan gravy | Recipe Renovator

11. Stir in the remaining stock, and turn up the heat until it starts to boil. You'll need to continue stirring to break up any clumps of roux, but they will dissolve into the soon-to-be gravy. There are some bits of turkey skin and meat in this photo.

12. How to make turkey pan gravy | Recipe Renovator

13. Continue cooking until thickened, about five minutes. Add black pepper if desired. I stop when the gravy is thick enough to hold open spaces in the bottom of the pan as I'm stirring, as in the photo.

Prep Time: 10 Minutes

Cook Time: 15 Minutes

Servings: 2

Ingredients

- 8 ounces cod Alaska cod, halibut, or tilapia, thawed overnight in refrigerator, patted very dry
- 8 ounces potatoes russet or Yukon gold, cut into matchsticks
- 1/4 cup all-purpose flour (gluten-free)
- 1/4 tsp sea salt omit for low-sodium, Menieres, migraine diets
- 1/4 tsp black pepper
- 1/4 tsp garlic powder
- 1/2 cup water (filtered or spring) or plain sparkling water

Tartar Sauce:

- 1/4 cup mayonnaise
- 1 lemon zest only (reserve lemon juice for another use)

- 1 tbsp pickle relish
- 1 tbsp pickle juice from sweet pickles
- 1 tbsp dill (fresh) finely snipped

Instructions

1. Soak the cut potatoes in water until ready to use, then drain and pat dry thoroughly with a clean kitchen towel.
2. Pat the fish fillets very dry and cut into smaller pieces if necessary for your air fryer space.
3. Whisk together the flour, spices, and water in a medium bowl until smooth. It should be very thin.
4. Preheat the air fryer to 400°F. Spray the basket well with olive oil or coconut oil spray.
5. Drop the potatoes into the basket, spritzing them with oil and tossing them to coat evenly. Sprinkle with additional salt (if using) and pepper.
6. Dip the fish fillets into the batter, allowing the excess to drip off. Place on the shelf in the basket above the potatoes.
7. Place the basket in air fryer and turn on to 400°F for 10 minutes.
8. Tartar sauce

9. Whisk together ingredients, starting with 1 tablespoon sweet pickle juice. Add more pickle juice if needed to get the consistency you want. Note that tartar sauce is not suitable for low-sodium, migraine, or Meniere's diets.

10. Serve fish and chips immediately with tartar sauce on the side.

Prep Time: 15 Minutes

Cook Time: 35 Minutes

Servings: 4

Ingredients

- 1 cup all-purpose flour (gluten-free) sifted (I recommend Bob's Red Mill 1 to 1)
- 1 tsp baking powder sifted to remove lumps
- 1/2 tsp granulated sugar (organic)
- 1/4 tsp sea salt
- 1/4 cup milk whole (organic if possible), warmed
- 1 tbsp milk whole (organic if possible), warmed
- 1 tbsp vegetable shortening I use Spectrum Organic, but Crisco or lard can be used.
- 2 eggs separated into four bowls (1 white per bowl, 1 yolk per bowl)
- 1 cup Monterey jack cheese grated

Instructions

1. Preheat the oven to 350°F. Prepare a baking sheet with fresh parchment paper that is lightly oiled or greased.

2. Whisk the flour, baking powder, sugar, and salt together.

3. Heat the milk (1/4 cup plus 1 tablespoon) and vegetable shortening in a microwave-safe bowl on medium-low power until the milk is warm and the shortening is melted.

4. Stir one egg yolk into the flour mixture, then add the warm milk a little at a time, mixing until you have a soft, pliable dough.

5. Let dough rest, covered, for 20 minutes. (This is critical for the dough to hydrate and not crack.)

6. Beat one egg white until very dry and stiff peaks form. Mix in the grated cheese with a spatula just until combined. Set aside.

7. Place the dough in the center of the oiled parchment paper and form it into a rough rectangle with your hands. If the dough feels dry or is cracking, add 1 teaspoon milk and work it into the dough. Cover the dough with plastic wrap, then roll out thinly into a

rectangle, resetting the plastic wrap as needed. You may have to pull the parchment flat.

8. Peel off the plastic wrap, then cut the dough into 4 rectangles with a knife. Place one-quarter of the cheese-egg white mixture in the center of each rectangle. Use a flat knife, thin spatula, or bench scraper to separate the edge of the dough from the parchment as you lift that edge. The goal is to fold it over like an envelope and lightly crimp the edges. Repeat to make the other rollos.

9. Beat the last egg yolk lightly with a fork, then brush the tops of each rollo with egg yolk. (You will have one egg white left over to use for another recipe. Do NOT be tempted to use both egg whites with the cheese in this recipe, as it will overfill the rollo.)

10. Bake for 35 minutes until the rollos are puffed and golden brown and the underside is golden and sounds hollow when tapped.

11. Eat as soon as they are cool enough to handle.